Healing Journey:

How I Overcame Endometriosis in 6 Weeks

By

Susan J. Derek

Healing Journey:

How I Overcame Endometriosis in 6 Weeks

Copyright © 2023 by Susan J. Derek

Table of Contents

Abstract

"'Healing Journey:'" The author's book, "How I Overcame Endometriosis in Six Weeks," is a very personal account of her battle with endometriosis and the life-changing journey she took to regain her health and well-being. Endometriosis, a long-term condition that affects millions of people worldwide, frequently causes debilitating pain, emotional difficulties, and concerns about fertility. The author provides readers with a path through the complexities of this condition based on her own experiences.

The book starts by giving an intensive comprehension of endometriosis, its side effects, and the significance of early conclusion. From the moment she first noticed symptoms to her decision to take control of her health, the author describes her own journey. A holistic treatment plan that incorporates the efficacy of nutrition, complementary therapies, and modifications to one's lifestyle is presented to the reader in a manner that is both clear and practical.

Readers will find the meaning of rest, sleep, and stress management in managing endometriosis side effects. The author discusses the crucial role that both in-person and online support networks play in the healing process in addition to advocating for professional guidance in the field of healthcare.

The core of the book lies in the writer's very own 6-week change, offering a substantial illustration of what is reachable with commitment and the right methodology. Readers are encouraged to adjust their timelines and establish individual goals as they progress through their own healing journey.

'Healing Journey: How I Overcame Endometriosis in 6 Weeks,' concludes by stressing the significance of reflection and long-term maintenance and by recognizing small victories. Examples of meal plans, recipes, guided meditation practices, and a template for a symptom diary are among the useful resources in the book.

The goal of this motivational and instructive guide is to give people who have endometriosis the tools they need to take control of their health, make well-informed choices, and find hope in the process of healing. By sharing her own way to recuperation, the creator offers an encouraging sign to those confronting the difficulties of endometriosis, advising them that change is conceivable, slowly and deliberately."

Introduction:

In quiet times of our lives, unexpected difficulties may arise that have a lasting impact on our journey. Endometriosis, a mysterious and frequently painful condition that affects millions of people worldwide, is one such obstacle. It is a condition which may affect our hopes and dreams as well as the day to day lives of us. I realize this very well since I've strolled the twisting road of endometriosis, exploring its exciting bends in the road, sympathizing with its aggravation, and eventually tracking down my approach to mending.

"Healing Journey: How I Overcame Endometriosis in 6 Weeks," is a heartfelt account of my own battle with endometriosis and the path I took to recovery. I'm telling my story not as a promise of quick fixes for everyone, but as a demonstration of the strength of the human spirit and the transformative power of determination, knowledge, and holistic approaches to healing.

Endometriosis is a condition that frequently leaves people feeling separated, misjudged, and overpowered by the mind-boggling trap of side effects and medicines. I'm hoping that by sharing my journey, I'll be able to give advice, motivation, and hope to those who are dealing with endometriosis or supporting a loved one through it.

In the following pages, you will be taken through my personal experiences, from the first time I noticed symptoms to the day I realized I was on the road to recovery. We're going to look at different parts of endometriosis, including its side effects, determination, and standard treatment choices, but we're also going to explore the universe of comprehensive healing, nourishment, care for ourselves, and the mind-blowing effect of constant organization.

I invite you to join me on this journey, whether you have just been diagnosed, have been battling endometriosis for a long time, or just want to learn more about the difficulties endometriosis sufferers face. We will discuss the methods and mental shifts that helped me alleviate my endometriosis symptoms in just six weeks. Your way might vary, yet realize that you are in good company, and recuperating is conceivable.

We can embrace the possibilities of a brighter, pain-free future with hope, determination, and a holistic approach. Let the journey to healing begin.

Chapter 1

Understanding Endometriosis in Simple Terms

Endometriosis is like a maze that many people, particularly women, may not fully comprehend. It's not an easy thing to deal with; however, the most important phase in managing it is to comprehend what it is.

What Is Endometriosis?

Imagine your body as a house, and inside this house is a special room called the uterus. Every month, this room gets ready for a possible guest, which is a fertilized egg. The room gets cleaned up and starts over if no one is there. This is your monthly period.

Now comes the difficult part. For some individuals, such as those with endometriosis, pieces of that particular room—such as wallpaper or carpet—start to appear outside the house, in other rooms, or even far from the house.

It's like these pieces are causing trouble. They can ache in the stomach or cause severe cramps, especially during the month (your period) when the room needs to be cleaned. They can also make it harder for people who want to have children to do so.

Common Signs and Challenges

People with endometriosis often experience problems like:

- discomfort in the abdomen, particularly during periods.
- Sex-related pain
- difficulty getting pregnant
- enduring constant fatigue.
- stomach upset or difficulty going to the bathroom.

Endometriosis, on the other hand, is like a sneaky guest who doesn't stay in the right room and causes all kinds of pains and discomfort.

Diagnosing Endometriosis

Specialists can see whether somebody has endometriosis by getting some information about their side effects and doing a few extraordinary tests. These tests might use pictures from a machine or a tiny camera to peek inside the belly—don't worry, it doesn't hurt much—to see what's going on.

Once doctors are certain that the condition is endometriosis, they can help the patient manage it and feel better.

So, in layman's terms, endometriosis is when parts of a special room in the body wander away from where they belong, resulting in pain and other issues. However, do not be concerned; there are strategies for overcoming it, and you are not alone on this journey.

Endometriosis not an easy thing to deal with; however, the most important phase in managing it is to comprehend what it is.

Chapter 2

My Journey Begins

I'll talk more about the early stages of my endometriosis journey in this chapter. Crucial points in my experience included realizing that I needed to take action and comprehending how my symptoms first began to manifest.

The Beginning of the Symptoms

My experience with endometriosis began with a series of confusing and sometimes overwhelming symptoms. It's critical to perceive that these side effects can change broadly from one individual to another; however, I trust sharing my experience will resonate with the people who have confronted similar difficulties.

For me, the first sign was *pain*, a constant, agonizing pain with each menstrual cycle. It was more than just the usual discomfort that comes with menstruation; My lower abdomen was being hit hard by a sharp, deep pain. It became increasingly disruptive to my day-to-day life as I could not ignore it.

Perhaps you can identify with this pain or have experienced other typical endometriosis symptoms like:

Dysmenorrhea: severe menstrual cramps that prevented me from working, studying, or participating in activities.

Dyspareunia: Pain during sexual activity strained my relationships and made it difficult to get close.

Problems with the Gut: Gut distress, bulging, and sporadic solid discharges that frequently harmonized with my period.

Chronic Anxiety: a constant sense of exhaustion that persisted even when I thought I should be getting enough sleep.

Recognizing these side effects and associating them to a potential medical issue was a critical initial phase in my journey. When you don't feel right, it's important to listen to your body and get help.

The Defining moment

The moment I realized that I could no longer ignore my symptoms or simply bear the pain was the turning point in my journey. It was time to find relief and answers.

In the beginning, I reached out to my closest friends and family to express my difficulties and seek emotional support. It was incredible how their understanding and support uplifted my spirits and gave me the courage to act.

The subsequent stage was to talk with a doctor — a fundamental choice that I need to stress. In this journey, your doctor is your ally, and they have the knowledge and tools to help you understand your body.

My doctor listened to my symptoms and concerns during my initial visit. They performed a physical examination and discussed potential diagnostic tests. In many cases, healthcare providers will conduct tests such as ultrasounds or X-ray outputs to get a superior look inside your body.

Keep in mind that talking to a doctor about your symptoms is an important first step toward controlling endometriosis. I encourage you to take this step and seek professional guidance if you haven't already.

Setting Realistic Expectations

The significance of setting realistic expectations for my journey was something else that I quickly realized. I was aware that it might take time to find a solution and ease my suffering, and I was eager to do so.

Endometriosis is a complicated condition that often requires long-term treatment. It's not about finding a quick fix; rather, it's about coming up with an all-encompassing strategy to boost your quality of life. I realized I should have been patient and determined in my quest for help.

Keep in mind that your journey may differ from mine as you continue along this journey, and that's perfectly acceptable. The most important point is that you are already on the right path to effectively managing endometriosis by recognizing your symptoms, seeking professional assistance, and setting realistic expectations.

Despite the unique challenges you face, your journey is full of opportunities for healing and growth.

Here are some ways I adopted when setting realistic expectations along this horrible journey

Educating Myself: I started by learning about endometriosis for myself. It was essential to comprehend the condition's chronic nature, common symptoms, and treatment options. I came to realize that symptom management was a more realistic goal and that endometriosis might not have a quick or permanent cure.

Seeking Professional Guidance: Endometriosis-specific healthcare professionals were consulted by me. They helped me set realistic expectations and gave me valuable insights into the condition. They explained that while treatments might make symptoms go away, they might not completely get rid of them, and it might take some time to figure out what works best for me.

Observing My Body: I learned to pay close attention to the signals sent by my body. I recorded my levels of pain, energy, and how different treatments or changes to my lifestyle affected me in a symptom diary. I was able to see patterns and alter my expectations based on how my body responded as a result of this.

Managing Expectations from the Heart: Emotional management was just as important as physical symptoms management. I knew that there would be good days as well as bad days. I avoided becoming discouraged when

I encountered setbacks and celebrated even small improvements as victories because I accepted this.

Setting Flexible Goals: I set flexible, achievable goals for myself. Instead of aiming for complete pain elimination, I focused on reducing the severity and frequency of my symptoms. These smaller, attainable goals allowed me to maintain a positive outlook and stay motivated.

Developing an Adaptive Mentality: I was happy to be flexible and open to trying different treatments. I had to be willing to try new approaches and adjust my strategies as needed because I knew that what worked for others might not work for me.

Establishing a Support System: I had a supportive group of friends and family who knew what it was like to have endometriosis. Their consolation and sympathy assisted me with keeping a practical viewpoint and offered close to home help during testing times.

Remaining Informed: I stayed up to date on new research and treatments for endometriosis. Because of this, I was able to have well-informed discussions with my healthcare providers and investigate new options that might be compatible with my objectives.

Practicing Self-Compassion: I stopped blaming myself and learned to be kind to myself. Endometriosis is not my fault, and managing it is a journey that calls for self-compassion and patience. I recognized that I was doing all that could be expected in light of the current situation.

Observing Little Wins: Every little improvement in my health was celebrated. Whether it was a day with less agony, expanded energy, or the capacity to participate in a movement I delighted in, perceiving these accomplishments assisted me with remaining spurred and keep an uplifting perspective.

When you don't feel right, it's important to listen to your body and get help.

Chapter 3

The Power of Nutrition

During my struggle to overcome endometriosis, one of the most important insights I gained was the significant impact that nutrition can have on managing the condition. This chapter delves into the crucial role that nutrition plays in the management of endometriosis and how making well-informed dietary choices can benefit your health.

The Relationship Between Diet and Endometriosis

Imagine that your body is like a finely tuned machine, and the fuel you give it affects how well it works. This fuel is nutrition, and it can help or hinder your body's ability to effectively manage endometriosis.

It is essential to comprehend the connection between endometriosis and diet. While explicit dietary decisions won't fix endometriosis, they can fundamentally affect your side effects and overall quality of life.

Foods to Include and Avoid

1. ***Anti-Inflammatory Foods***: Inflammation is a vital driver of endometriosis-related torment and uneasiness. Inflammation can be reduced by including foods that reduce inflammation in your diet. Some of these foods are:

- Fruits and vegetables (berries, salad greens, turmeric): brimming with anti-inflammatory antioxidants.
- Oats, brown rice, and other whole grains: Reduce inflammation and support gut health with fiber and nutrients.

2. ***Omega 3 Fatty Acids:*** Inflammation may be reduced through the presence of these fatty acids in fish. Think about adding fish into your diet or using Omega 3 supplements, based on the advice of your doctor.

3. ***Foods rich in fiber:*** In support of digestive health and regular bowel movements, eating foods high in fiber can help reduce gastrointestinal symptoms that are often associated with endometriosis.

4. ***Lean proteins:*** including protein from lean sources such as beans, tofu and poultry is important to maintain a healthy body for the necessary amino acids.

5. ***Dairy Alternatives:*** A few people with endometriosis find that dairy products or milk worsen their symptoms. You may want to experiment with coconut yogurts or almonds, if you feel that you might be allergic to milk.

On the other hand, certain dietary habits and foods can make endometriosis symptoms worse. Some examples include:

1. ***Processed Foods:*** Foods that have been highly processed and are frequently packed with sugars and unhealthy fats can exacerbate pain and inflammation.

2. ***Alcohol and caffeine:*** Drinking too much alcohol and caffeine can make it hard to sleep and make hormonal imbalances worse, which could make endometriosis symptoms worse.

3. ***Red Meat:*** Increased inflammation has been linked to a high intake of red meat, particularly processed meats.

4. ***Gluten:*** A gluten-free diet has been shown to improve symptoms in some endometriosis sufferers. Gluten responsiveness can intensify gastrointestinal issues.

Recipes and Meal Planning

A proactive approach to managing endometriosis is to devise a meal plan based on your dietary preferences and symptoms. The following is how you can begin:

1. ***Talk to a nutritionist:*** Think about speaking with a registered dietitian who specializes in managing endometriosis. They can assist you in creating a bespoke, goal-oriented meal plan.

2. ***Healthy Meals:*** Aim for balanced meals that incorporate a variety of nutrient-dense foods. Include plenty of colorful fruits and vegetables as well as protein-rich and healthy fats.

3. ***Control of Size:*** To avoid discomfort-causing overeating, pay attention to portion sizes. If you have digestive issues, eating smaller meals more frequently may be beneficial.

4. ***Stay hydrated:*** Satisfactory hydration is pivotal. Limit sugary and caffeinated beverages and drink more water and herbal teas.

5. ***Mindful Nutrition***: Eat mindfully by taking your time, listening to your body's signals of hunger and fullness, and avoiding distractions while you eat.

During my struggle to overcome endometriosis, one of the most important insights I gained was the significant impact that nutrition can have on managing the condition.

Chapter 4

Approaches to Holistic Healing

My journey to recovery from endometriosis included more than just dietary changes and conventional treatments. I also discovered the transformative power of holistic healing approaches, which supplemented my general system for dealing with this mind-boggling condition. In this chapter, I'll share how these all-encompassing or holistic practices became vital to my well-being and how they could help you as well.

Complementary Therapies: A Holistic View

Complementary therapies are methods that complement traditional medicine to improve one's overall health and well-being. Although they may not directly treat endometriosis, they can greatly enhance your quality of life by addressing symptoms and assisting your body's natural healing processes.

Yoga: Embracing Mind-Body Connection

Yoga was a distinct advantage in my journey with endometriosis. Its gentle yet powerful postures, profound breathing activities, and mindfulness techniques helped me in many ways:

- Management of Pain: Menstrual pain and pelvic discomfort can be alleviated in certain yoga poses. My mobility has been improved and the severity of my cramps reduced by regular practice.

- Stress Management: Yoga promotes unwinding and diminishes pressure, which is vital on the grounds that pressure can intensify endometriosis side effects. I was able to cultivate a sense of calm that had a positive effect on my overall well-being by incorporating yoga into my routine.

- Mind-Body Connection: Yoga made me more connected to my body. This allowed me to study the signals I was receiving from my body with more detail, taking care of myself and responding accordingly.

Meditation: Finding Inner Peace

Meditation has been an integral part of my holistic healing arsenal. Two aspects of meditation that could benefit from a variety of ways are mindfulness and focused attention:

- Pain Management: Endometriosis-related pain can be alleviated by activating the body's natural pain-relief mechanisms through meditation.

- Stress Management: Ongoing torment and stress frequently remain inseparable. I was able to manage my stress and lessen its impact on my symptoms by using meditation techniques like guided imagery and deep breathing.

- Sleep Improvement: Sleep problems plague many people with endometriosis. Meditation can improve the quality of your sleep, allowing your body to heal and recover more quickly.

Acupuncture:

Acupuncture, a form of traditional Chinese medicine, involves inserting fine needles into specific body points to regulate the flow of qi, or energy, throughout the body. Despite my initial skepticism, I discovered that acupuncture was surprisingly effective:

- Reduction of Pain: My pelvic pain and menstrual cramps were significantly reduced during acupuncture sessions. It appeared to upgrade the body's normal relief from discomfort instruments.

- Regulation of Hormones: Acupuncture may help people with endometriosis-related hormonal imbalances by regulating hormones, according to some studies.

- Stress Reduction: Sessions of acupuncture helped people feel more relaxed and less stressed, which improved their overall health.

Exercise: Taking Care of Your Physical Health

Regular exercise was an important part of my holistic approach to managing my endometriosis. There are many advantages to exercise which you know, a whole lot:

- Management of Pain: Endorphins, the body's natural painkillers, were released when people did low-impact exercises like swimming or walking to help reduce pain.

- Stress Management: Exercise can significantly reduce stress. When you're dealing with a chronic condition, physical activity can help you feel more at ease and mentally strong.

- Hormone Balance: Maintaining a healthy weight through exercise may help balance hormones which was really helpful for me.

I was able to experience a more significant reduction in endometriosis symptoms and an overall improvement in my quality of life by incorporating these holistic healing approaches into my daily routine. These practices furnished me with a feeling of strengthening and self-care that supplemented traditional clinical medicines and dietary changes. Keep in mind that no two people's journeys are the same, so look into these holistic approaches with an open mind and seek advice from medical professionals when necessary.

Complementary therapies can greatly enhance your quality of life by addressing symptoms and assisting your body's natural healing processes.

Chapter 5

The Importance of Rest and Sleep

We will discuss a crucial aspect of my struggle to overcome endometriosis in this chapter: the significance of adequate sleep and rest. You'll find practical steps I took that not only made my symptoms go away but also made my mind and body feel better. Therefore, let's set out on this journey together, with the expectation of better sleep and brighter days to come.

The Power of Restorative Sleep

Consider sleep to be the body's reset button, a time when it repairs, reenergizes, and rejuvenates itself. Sadly, many people with endometriosis have trouble sleeping, which can make other symptoms worse. My journey toward better rest started with a comprehension of its essential job in managing endometriosis.

Step 1: Prioritizing Sleep

The first step was straightforward but profound: I put my sleep first. This required realizing that getting enough sleep was not a luxury; It played a crucial role in my recovery. I made a promise to sleep for the recommended 7 to 9 hours each night.

Step 2: Creating a Restful Environment

The next logical step was to create an environment that was conducive to sleep. I made my bedroom a haven for relaxation:

Darkness: My blackout curtains helped me regulate my circadian rhythm by keeping my room dark at night.

Comfort: I became best friends with a comfortable bed and pillows. The quality of your sleep can be significantly affected by the appropriate support.

Zone Devoid of Technology: I banned blue-light-emitting screens from my bedroom, which can disrupt sleep patterns, as a technology-free zone.

Relaxing with Music: I learned how effective calm; gentle music is for relieving stress. I was able to relax and create a peaceful atmosphere in my sleeping space by playing soft, peaceful music before going to bed.

Temperature Management: To get a good night's sleep, it was important to keep the temperature of the room comfortable—not too hot or too cold.

Step 3: Establishing a Sleep Routine

Consistency in a sleep routine is the key to getting a good night's sleep. I laid out a rest routine by heading to sleep and awakening at similar times consistently, even on weekends. My body's internal clock was regulated by this, making it easier to fall asleep and get up refreshed.

Step 4: Wind-Down Rituals

As the time for bed drew near, I began incorporating some calming wind-down rituals:

Reading: Taking part in a quieting movement like perusing a book helped sign to my body that the time had come to unwind.

Warm Bath: A warm shower before bed can loosen up tense muscles and advance a feeling of peacefulness.

Step 5: Keeping away from Rest Disruptors

Certain propensities and substances can disturb rest. I did whatever it takes to limit their effect:

Alcohol and caffeine: In the hours leading up to bedtime, I stayed away from alcohol and caffeine.

Heavy Meals: I had my last meal a few hours before going to bed because heavy or spicy meals can make it hard to sleep.

Screen Time: I restricted my use of screens at night, particularly smartphones and computers, which emit blue light that can hinder the body's production of hormones that induce sleep.

I not only saw an improvement in my sleep but also a significant decrease in the symptoms associated with endometriosis as a result of taking these practical steps. A very much refreshed body and psyche are strong partners in the battle against this condition. You can rest assured that you can achieve better sleep and a brighter, less painful future by incorporating these strategies into your daily routine as you move forward on your journey. In the next chapter, we'll explore the importance of seeking professional help and the various treatment options available for managing endometriosis.

Consider sleep to be the body's reset button, a time when it repairs, reenergizes, and rejuvenates itself.

Chapter 6

Seeking Professional Help

One of the most important steps I took on my journey to manage endometriosis was to seek professional assistance. This chapter emphasizes the significance of speaking with endometriosis-specific healthcare providers, discussing my symptoms, and investigating various treatment options. I hope to inspire you to seek the advice of medical professionals by sharing my personal experiences.

The Power of a Healthcare Team

When dealing with a complex condition like endometriosis, I realized that I needed a healthcare team that could give me the knowledge and direction I needed to manage it well. Here's how I established this crucial support network:

- ***Finding the Right Healthcare Provider***

The journey started by tracking down a compassionate and educated essential healthcare provider. I sought recommendations from companions, family, and online care groups, which assisted me with distinguishing medical care experts experienced in endometriosis care.

I made an appointment to talk about my symptoms and concerns once I found the right doctor. It was vital to find somebody who viewed my side effects in a serious way and was able to investigate treatment choices custom-made to my necessities.

- ***Consultation with Specialists***

Endometriosis frequently involves problems with digestion, pain management, and gynecological health. As a result, I sought advice from professionals who could deal with every aspect of my condition:

Gynecologist: My care was centered on a seasoned gynecologist who offered advice on how to deal with menstrual symptoms, fertility issues, and hormonal treatments.

Specialist in managing pain: Endometriosis can be associated with significant levels of chronic pain. I was able to investigate various medications and methods of pain relief that were tailored to my condition after consulting with a specialist in pain management.

Gastroenterologist: A gastroenterologist can provide helpful insights and treatment options if you experience gastrointestinal symptoms like bloating, discomfort in the bowels, or constipation.

Nutritionist/Dietitian: I saw an endometriosis-focused registered dietitian to improve my diet for symptom management. They helped me make well-informed dietary decisions thanks to their guidance.

- *Networks of Support*

Endometriosis can be a difficult emotional journey, and I needed to find support networks for my well-being:

Endometriosis Support Groups: I felt a sense of community through the internet and local support groups. It was incredibly comforting to share my experiences, advice and emotional support with other people who understood what I went through.

Health care professional: Mental well-being can be affected by endometriosis. I was able to develop coping mechanisms and address any emotional difficulties that arose during my journey by consulting a mental health professional.

- *Advocating for Myself*

I've learned over the course of this process that it is necessary to advocate for myself. By asking questions, seeking second opinions if necessary and working with health care professionals in order to make informed decisions about the treatment plan for me, I have actively participated in taking care of myself.

- *Monitoring and Adjusting*

Endometriosis management is not static; It is fluid and may necessitate constant adjustments. My healthcare providers were able to monitor my progress, evaluate the efficacy of my treatment, and make any necessary adjustments to improve my care during my regular follow-up appointments.

By setting up networks and health care teams that supported me, I have gained access to a wealth of knowledge, resources and emotional support. I've learned that you don't have to tackle endometriosis alone; there are experts and communities ready to go with you.

I made an appointment to talk about my symptoms and concerns once I found the right doctor.

Chapter 7

Tracking Progress

Keeping track of your progress toward overcoming endometriosis is similar to using a map to navigate; You can see where you've been and where you're going with it. I will discuss the tools I used, the significance of monitoring your journey, and how these insights can empower you on your way to relief and recovery in this chapter.

The Journey Is a Marathon, not a Sprint

Endometriosis management is a long-term commitment, and if you don't see immediate results, it's easy to get discouraged. Tracking your progress helps with this. You can stay motivated and make well-informed decisions about your treatment plan by measuring your journey in concrete ways.

Creating a Progress Tracker

In my journey, creating a progress tracker was a crucial step. It allowed me to see how my health was changing over time in various ways. What I did was as follows:

Step 1: Identify Key Metrics

To begin, I identified key metrics that reflected my overall health and symptoms of endometriosis. Among these metrics were:

Levels of Pain: I was able to identify patterns and triggers when I rated my daily pain levels using a pain scale such as NRS, VDS VAS, etc.

Menstrual Symptoms: I was able to see if my menstrual symptoms, like cramps, bloating, and heavy bleeding, were getting better by keeping track of them.

Levels of energy: To see how well I was coping with fatigue, I kept track of my energy levels throughout the day.

Dietary Choices: Keeping a food journal assisted me with checking what my eating regimen meant for my side effects and whether dietary changes were having an effect.

Step 2: Choose a Method of Tracking

I chose the method of tracking that was most effective for me. Digital apps are preferred by some, while journals on paper are preferred by others. I utilized a mix of both:

Digital Software: I found it easy to use smartphone apps that track my habits and symptoms like symptom tracker, journal my health etc. They made it possible for me to quickly enter data and produce charts that were simple to read.

Paper Diary: Putting pen to paper has a certain satisfying quality. For more in-depth reflections and notes, I used a paper journal.

Step 3: Set a Tracking Schedule

When it comes to tracking progress, consistency is essential. I established a timetable for data entry. I was able to identify patterns and connections between various activities and metrics through daily tracking.

Analyzing the Data

As I continued to monitor my progress, I learned important lessons:

Identifying Triggers: Patterns emerged that assisted me identify potential triggers for symptom flare-ups. Some foods or levels of stress, for instance, seem to be associated with increased pain.

Treatment Viability: I was able to evaluate with objectivity whether treatments and changes in lifestyle were having a positive effect. I was able to have discussions with my healthcare team based on this information.

Empowerment: I was able to take an active role in my care because I could track my progress. I felt more in charge and could make adjustments to my treatment plan in view of information-driven knowledge.

Using Insights to Make Better Decisions

With the information from my progress tracker, I was able to work well with my healthcare team. Based on trends in my progress, we could talk about tweaks to my treatment, changes to my medication, or additional investigations.

Endometriosis is a journey that continues over time. By keeping tabs on your development, you're checking your side effects as well as acquiring significant bits of knowledge that engage you to come to informed conclusions about your wellbeing. Keep in mind that each data point brings you one step closer to relief and recovery as you continue your journey.

The Journey Is a Marathon, not a Sprint

Chapter 8

Embracing Every Step: Celebrating Small Victories

Endometriosis is a never-ending journey with unexpected detours and twists. In this part, we should investigate an alternate point of view — one that urges you to persevere as well as to flourish even with this perplexing condition. It's tied in with embracing each step of your journey and praising the little triumphs en route.

The Relentless Nature of Endometriosis

Endometriosis can frequently feel like an uphill battle. However, there are instances of triumph, perseverance, and personal development that merit recognition within this challenging season.

Reevaluating Progress: Little Triumphs Matter

It's fundamental to reevaluate how we view progress with regards to endometriosis. Consider that each small victory along the way is a significant achievement that merits celebration rather than solely focusing on the ultimate destination of complete relief. These triumphs are the venturing stones that drive you forward on your journey.

What Are Small Victories?
Small victories can take many different forms, and each person experiences them differently. Here are a few models:

A Day Free from Pain: Praise a day when your pain is more manageable or less serious than expected.

Participating in Pleasant exercises: If you are able to engage in an activity that you enjoy without being hindered by symptoms, it is a victory that deserves to be celebrated.

Improved Quality of Sleep: Upgrades in your rest examples can extraordinarily affect your general prosperity.

Managing symptoms successfully: It is a cause for celebration when a new treatment or lifestyle change results in a noticeable reduction in symptoms.

Mental and Profound Versatility: It is a significant personal accomplishment if you find that you are better able to deal with the emotional difficulties that come with endometriosis.

Why Celebrate Small Victories?
There are a number of important reasons to celebrate small victories:

Stimulates Motivation: Even if your progress is insignificant, acknowledging it can inspire you to keep moving forward. It reaffirms the possibility of positive change.

Enhances Adaptability: Resilience is cultivated when you acknowledge your capacity to overcome obstacles and setbacks. It builds up the conviction that you can explore the difficult times.

Enhances General Well-Being: Positive thinking can improve your mental and emotional health. It serves as a reminder that your condition alone does not define your life.

How to Celebrate Small Victories

The following are some ways to celebrate and remember your small victories:

Journaling: Keep a journal where you can record your daily progress and accomplishments.

Share with Friends and family: Share your triumphs with loved ones who figure out your journey and can celebrate with you.

Reward Yourself: As a reward for your accomplishments, treat yourself to something special.

Establish milestones: Celebrate when you reach milestones you've set. These can be present moment or long-haul objectives.

Reflect and Offer Thanks: Pause for a minute to ponder your journey and offer thanks for the headway you've made.

Motivate Others: Sharing your victories can give others who are going through the same things hope and inspiration.

Celebrate Your Strength and Embrace Your Journey

Endometriosis may present numerous challenges, but you have the strength to overcome them and the resilience to thrive. You can make your journey more fulfilling and empowering by focusing on the small victories rather than the difficulties. So, let's celebrate your incredible strength and take every small step in the right direction.

> *You can make your journey more fulfilling and empowering by focusing on the small victories rather than the difficulties.*

Chapter 9

My Transformation in 6 Weeks

I'd like to tell you about the amazing transformation I went through in just six weeks of focusing on endometriosis management. It was a time of remarkable progress and renewed optimism, but it also served as a crucial reminder that battling this complicated condition is unquestionably a marathon, not a sprint.

At the six-week mark of my endometriosis journey, I arrived at a huge defining moment. The progressions I had carried out — adjusting my eating regimen, consolidating comprehensive practices, and intently keeping tabs on my development — started to yield significant outcomes. The positive changes I saw astonished me.

My life was consumed by pain, exhaustion, and uncertainty prior to this journey. I had suffered from endometriosis for a number of years, denying me precious opportunities and moments. I had the impression that I was merely surviving and not truly living. However, I was unable to continue letting this crippling condition define me. As I committed to taking charge of my health, my determination grew.

After six weeks of consistent work, as described in the preceding chapters, I began to notice nudges of improvement. The pain began to get less frequent and more intense. I could get back into the things I used to do. I no longer felt enslaved by fatigue as my energy levels increased. The hope I had almost lost came back to life.

But things weren't always easy. I experienced days of frustration and discouragement. I reminded myself during these times that managing endometriosis is in fact a marathon, not a sprint. Even though progress was sluggish, it was still progress.

Not only did the six-week mark became a turning point in my journey, but also in my mindset. I came to the realization that I was in charge of my destiny and that this condition did not have to control me. The mix of a better eating routine, comprehensive practices, and tenacious following of my advancement had opened another part in my life.

I continued on this path with renewed resolve, eager to see what transformations lay ahead. Although endometriosis remained a part of my life for years, it no longer controlled or subdued me. I was prepared to run the marathon with endurance, strength, and the unwavering belief that I would have a better future with no trace of it.

Continuing the Journey...

As the weeks turned into months, I remained steadfast in my resolve to treat endometriosis. I was aware that this journey was not a short-term fix but rather a change in lifestyle. The underlying six weeks had given an establishment, however I expected to continue to accomplish enduring outcomes.

I discovered even more effective methods for managing endometriosis as I continued to adhere to my carefully constructed plan. I began consolidating specific herbs and supplements known for their anti-inflammatory properties into my daily routine (you can get it in my book *'THE 6-WEEK ENDO-DIET PLAN THAT CHANGED MY LIFE'* on Amazon). My diet and holistic practices were in sync with these natural remedies, which further reduced pain and inflammation.

I continued steadfast with the process that brought the significant improvement and more as revealed above and over the long run, I saw an exceptional change in my general well-being. My life became devoid of the agony that had once dominated it. During my darkest hours, I could engage in activities I had never considered. I felt more alive than I had in years, and my energy levels shot through the roof.

The change was more than just physical; It was also mental and emotional. I had overcome the feelings of helplessness and despair that had previously engulfed me. Every aspect of my life was influenced by my newly acquired sense of control and empowerment. I adopted a positive outlook, which enabled me to overcome obstacles with perseverance and optimism.

Endometriosis no longer overshadowed my life as time went on. It was as yet a piece of my set of experiences, however it at this point not characterized my present. Understanding that consistency was the key to preventing the condition, I continued living a healthy lifestyle.

I was thankful for the journey because it had not only healed my body but also changed my life as a whole. For those who are dealing with endometriosis, my story became a beacon of hope. I turned into a supporter, sharing my encounters and information to help those still amidst their battles.

I no longer feel the effects of endometriosis in my body today. A time in my life that taught me the value of resilience, determination, and self-care is now a distant memory. Knowing that I have reclaimed my life from the clutches of this complicated condition, I continue to treasure each day without pain.

My battle with endometriosis was, in fact, a marathon that I fought through with tenacity and unwavering devotion. I was not only healthier when I crossed the finish line, but my mind and spirit were also stronger. Furthermore, in doing as such, I demonstrated that with versatility and a balanced methodology, it's feasible to defeat even the most considerable of difficulties.

Endometriosis no longer overshadowed my life as time went on. It was as yet a piece of my set of experiences, however it at this point not characterized my present.

Chapter 10

Your Healing Journey

As you embark on your healing journey to overcome endometriosis, we will shift the focus of this final chapter from my journey to yours in this chapter. This chapter focuses on empowerment, self-discovery and accepting the possibilities in front of us.

Your Individual Journey

Endometriosis treatment is an individual journey. It's possible that what worked for me won't work exactly the same way for you. That's the beauty of your journey: it's a blank canvas on which you can write your own story about your unique experiences, triumphs, and challenges.

Setting Goals:

The first step is to set clear, attainable goals. What goals do you have for your journey to healing? Defining your objectives will give you direction and drive, whether it's to reduce pain, increase energy, or improve your overall well-being.

Building Your Support Network:

It is vital to have a solid support system. Visit support groups and consult medical professionals specialized in endometriosis, as well as your loved ones who understand what you're going through. Be surrounded by people who lift you up and give you hope.

Embracing Adaptability
Flexibility and adaptability are essential. Along the way, you might try different treatments, look into new ways to cope, and make adjustments. As you get a better understanding of what works best for you, be open to change and willing to change.

Keeping track of your progress and celebrating your victories
Much like my journey, yours will be full of challenges as well as victories. Keep an advancement tracker to screen your journey, celebrate little triumphs, and remain inspired. Recognize that even the smallest advances are significant.

Building Hope and Resilience
Your companion on this journey is resilience. Resilience enables you to rebound stronger from times of frustration and setbacks. During the more difficult times, cultivate hope and let it serve as your guiding light.

Remember that managing endometriosis is not a sprint but rather a marathon. In the short term, you might see progress, but the journey is on-going. Remain committed, remain tough, and remain confident.

Conclusion

Your Journey to Triumph Over Endometriosis

In conclusion, the fact that you were able to overcome endometriosis is evidence of your remarkable strength and resilience. The journey is marked by determination, adaptability and the unwavering hope. The path may be difficult, but it also offers numerous chances for personal development, transformation, and growth.

You've learned about the power of holistic approaches, the significance of self-care, and the significance of celebrating even the smallest victories throughout this book. You now know that managing endometriosis is a marathon, a journey that requires constant dedication and adaptability.

Keep in mind that your path to healing is unique as you begin it. It's okay if what works best for you is different from what works for others. Put forth clear objectives, fabricate areas of strength for an organization, and embrace flexibility as you investigate medicines and survival techniques.

Above all else, instill resilience and optimism. Resilience will enable you to rise stronger in the face of frustration and setbacks. Keep in mind the potential for mending, and never fail to focus on the expectation that lights your direction.

A tale of triumph, empowerment, and a brighter future awaits you on your journey. You are not on this journey alone. There is a local area of people, medical care suppliers, and friends and family prepared to help you constantly.

Now is the beginning of your healing journey, and I am absolutely certain that you will survive and triumph. As you overcome endometriosis, may your journey be filled with joy, strength, and transformation.